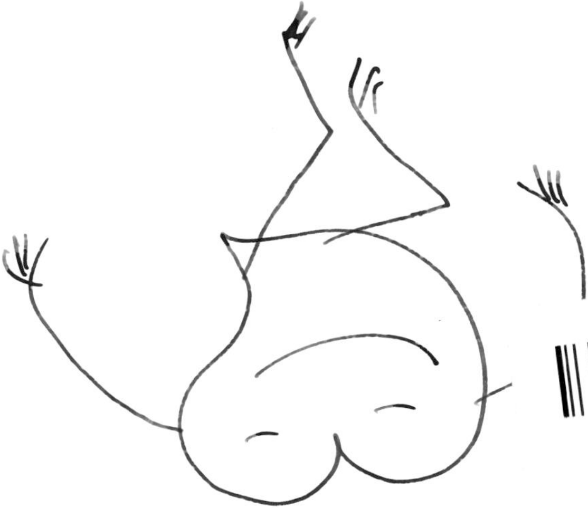

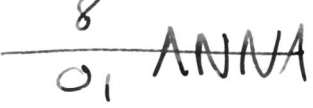

ANNAtomy

Cartoons
by
ANNA

1.–6. Tausend
Impressum:
© Anna R. Hartmann
annah@rtmann.ch
www.annahartmann.net
Druck Schwabe & Co. AG, Muttenz
Pharma Information with
Bergli Books AG, Basel, Switzerland
ISBN 3-905 252-03-1

"ANNAtomy" is a cartoon case history of Switzerland's health care system by ANNA, the well-known Swiss cartoonist. The protagonists are politicians, scientists, doctors, therapists, nurses and patients. For ANNAtomy ANNAtomizes not only the human body, but also the human psyche, exposing people's characters and the kinds of relationship which develop between patients, doctors and nursing staff.

ANNA's caricatures and cartoons appear in a number of Swiss and German newspapers and magazines and several collections of her works have been published as books.

"ANNAtomy" is the second publication of ANNA and the Pharma Information to be dedicated to patients, their organizations and self-help groups. Part of the proceeds from the sale of this book will go towards supporting the virtual patient platform www.patienten.ch as well as the work and advisory services of the patient groups it represents.

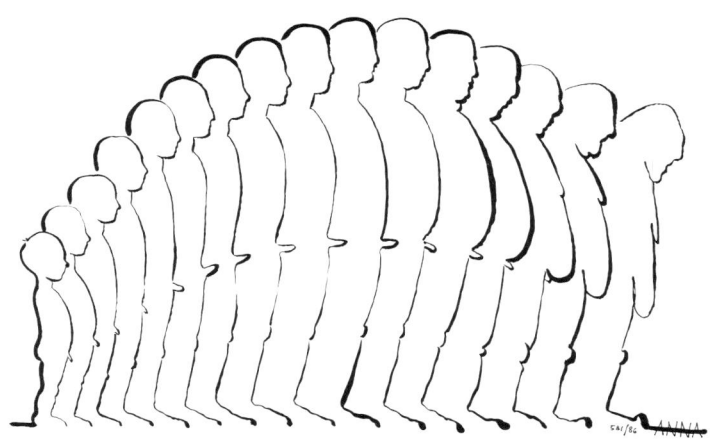

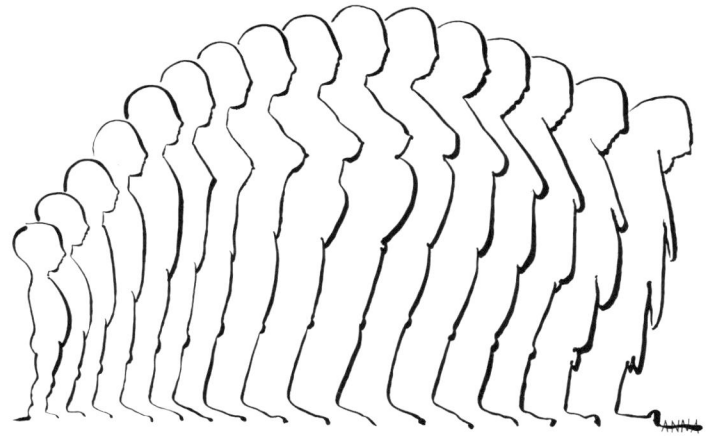

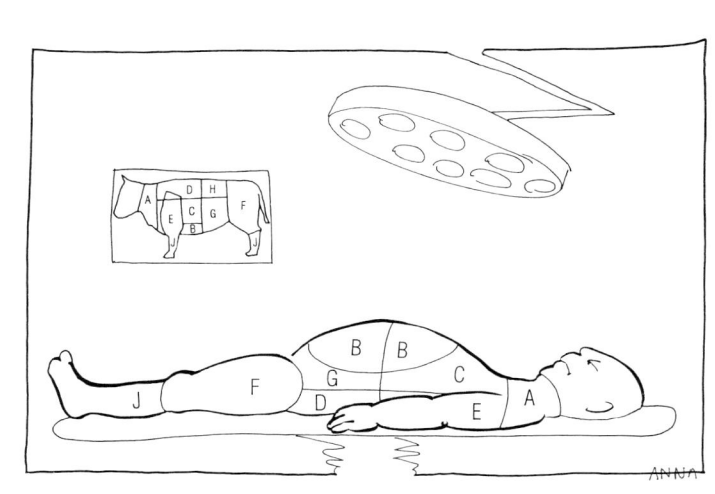

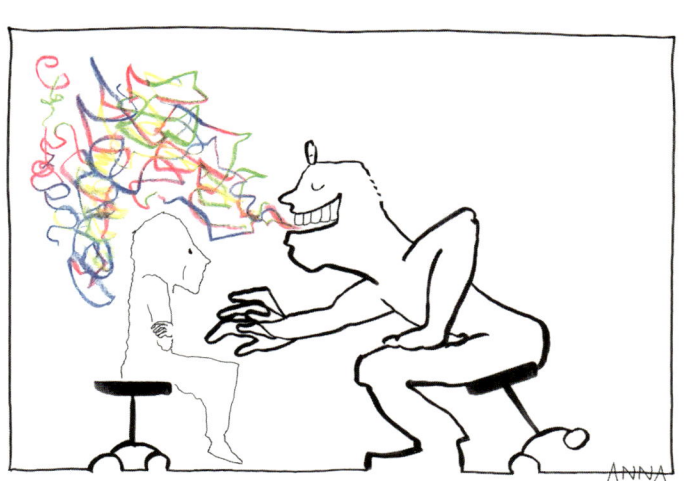

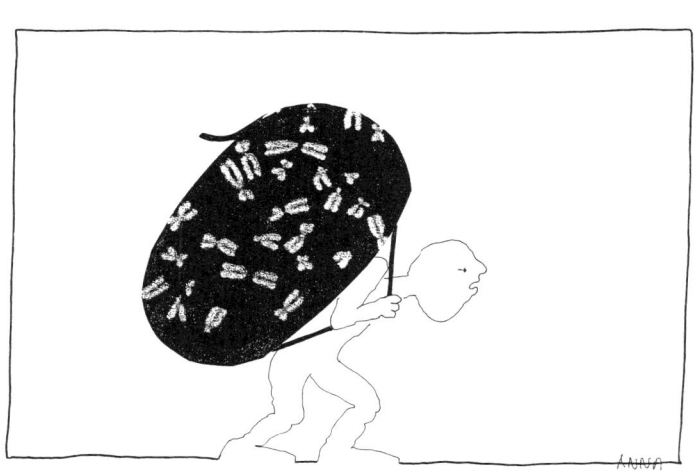

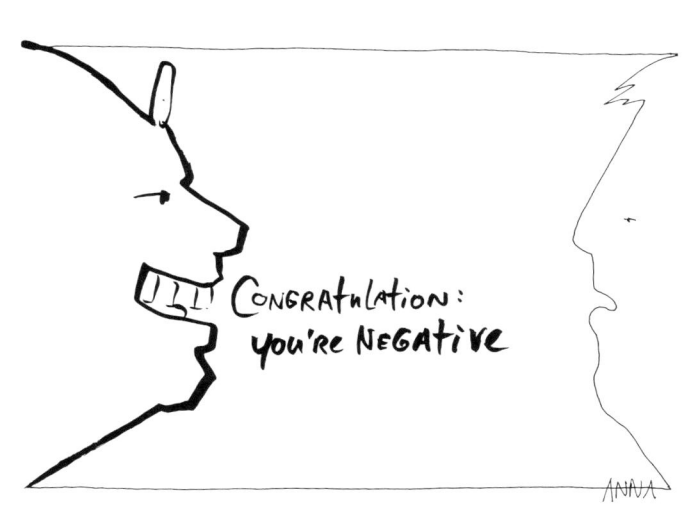

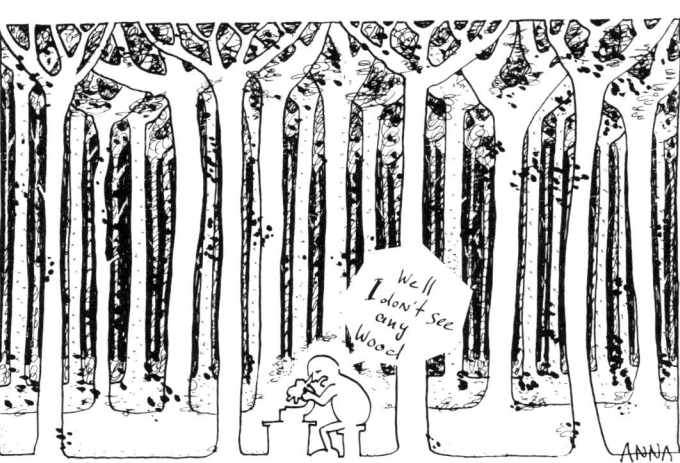

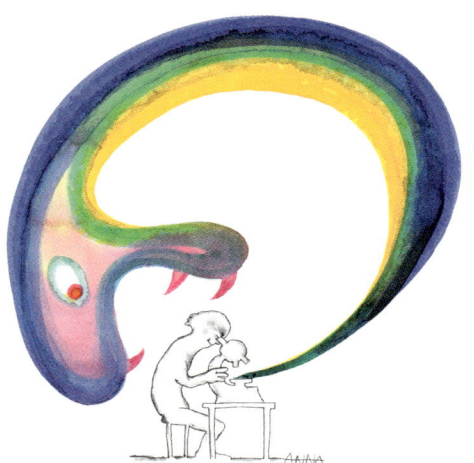

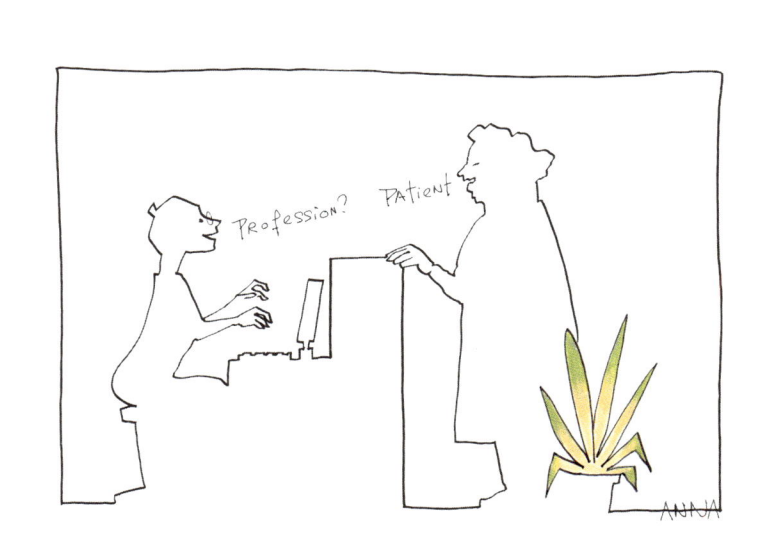

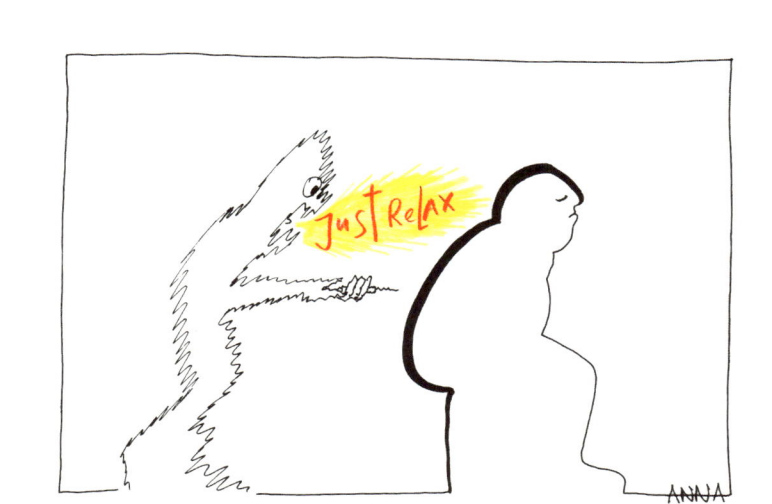

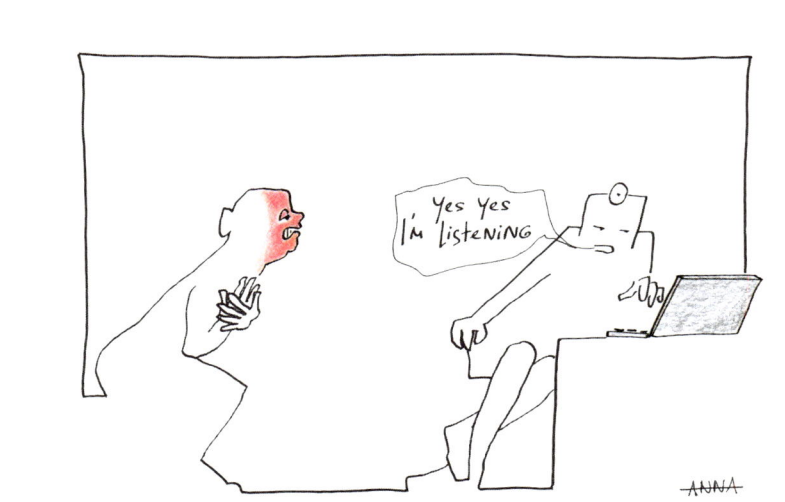

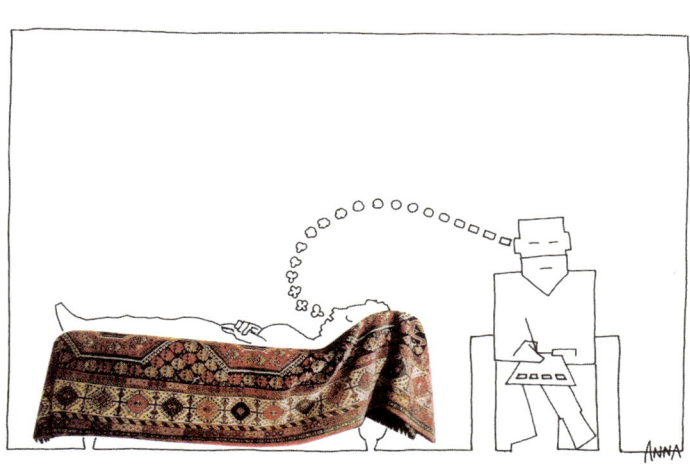

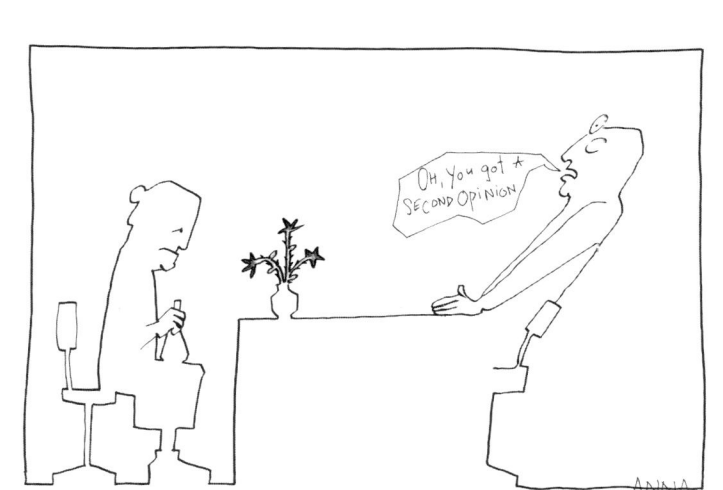

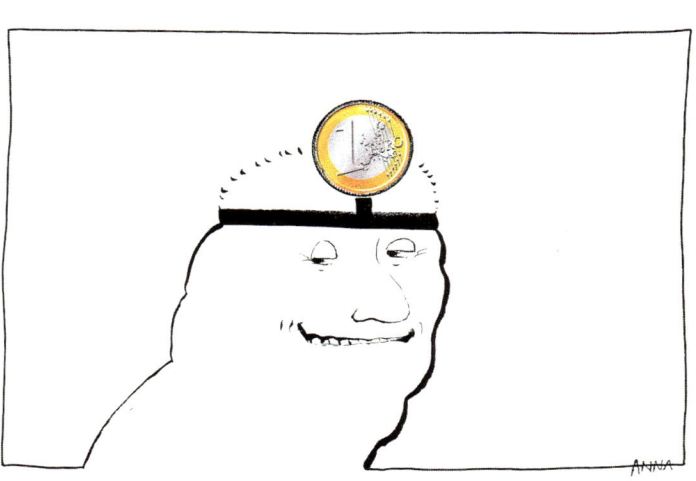

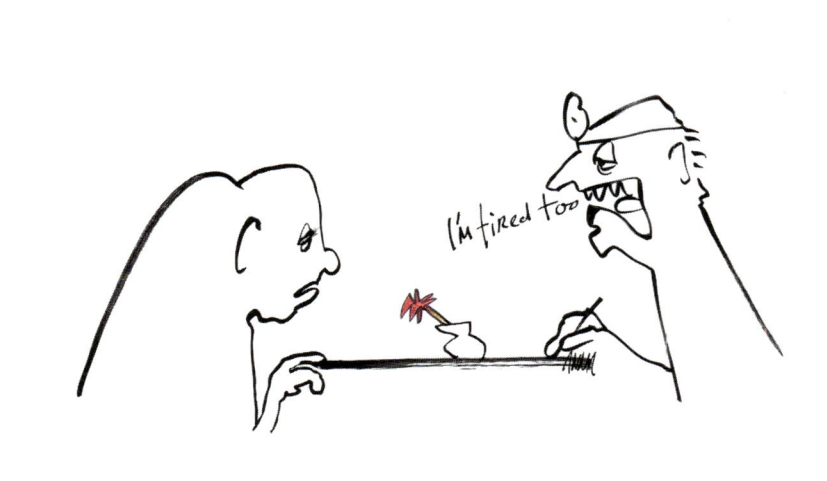

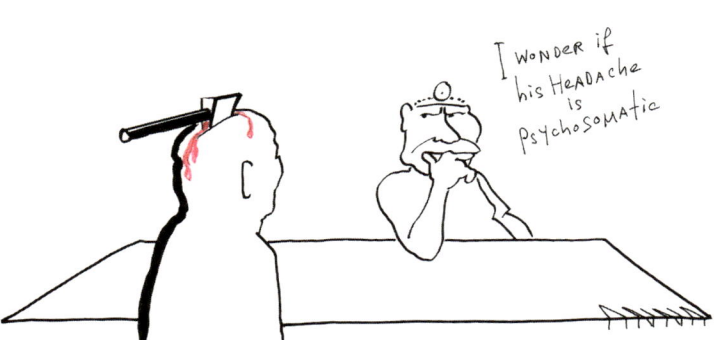

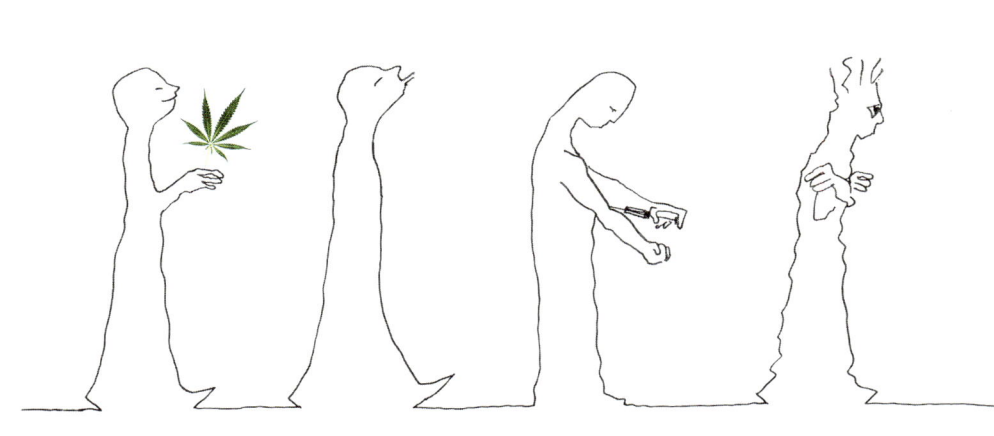

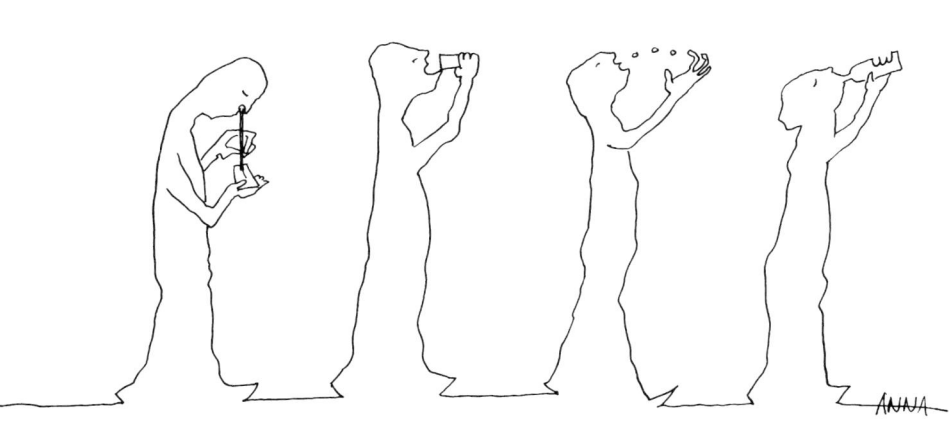

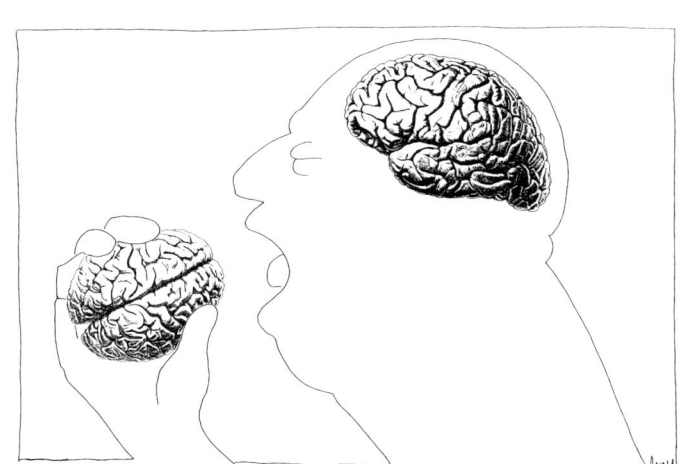

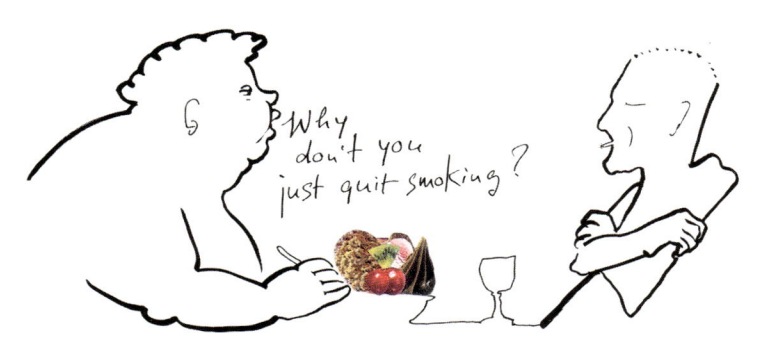

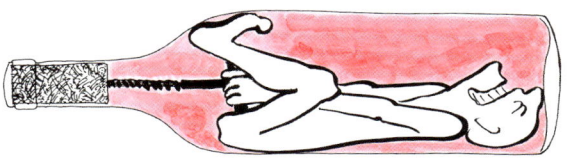

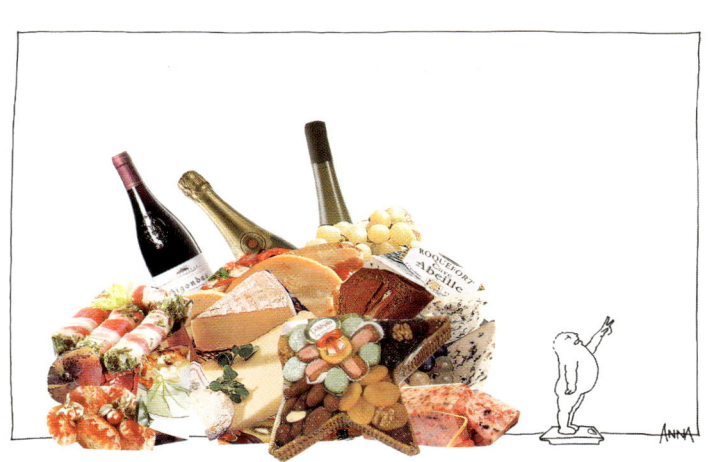

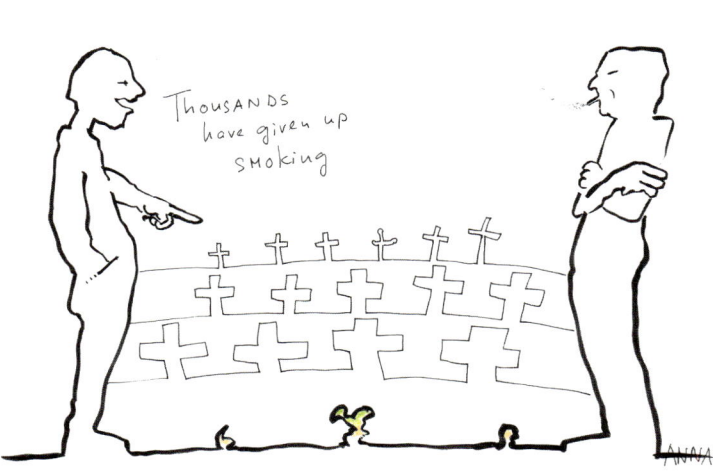

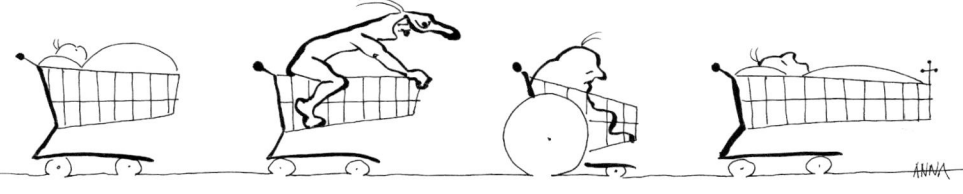

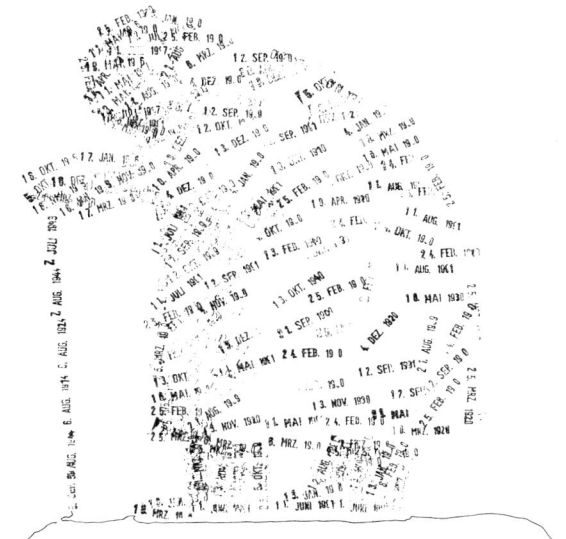

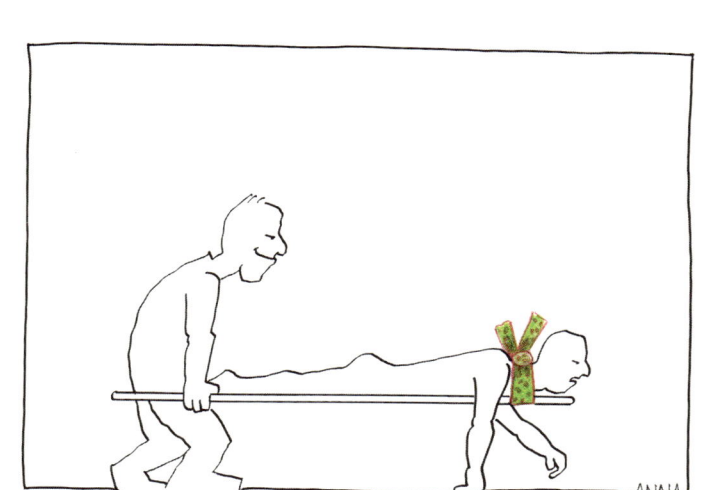

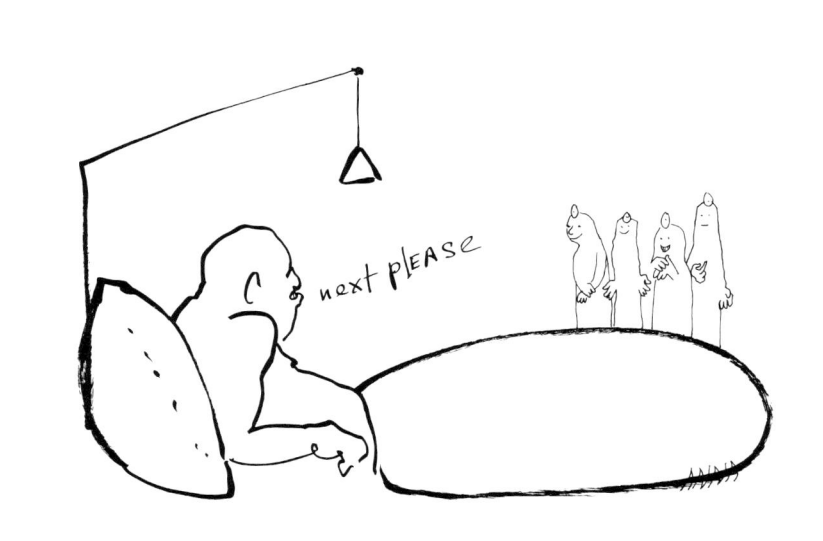

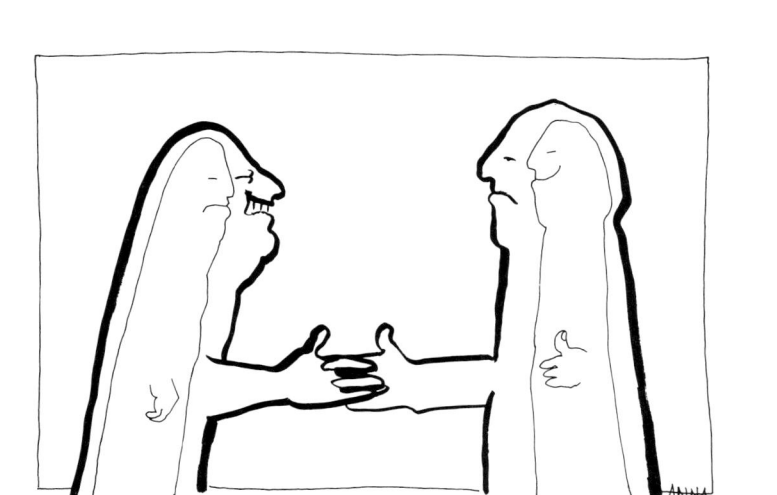

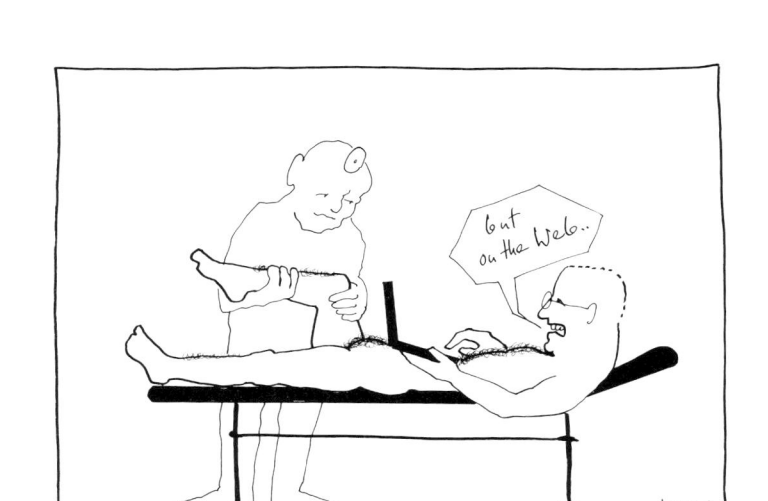

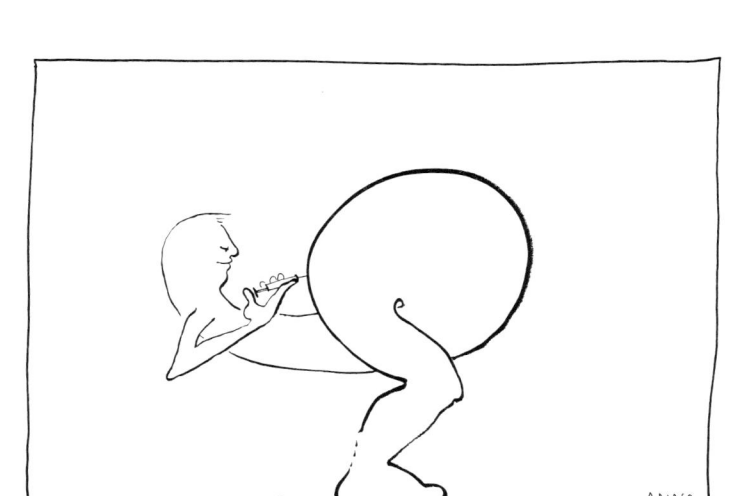

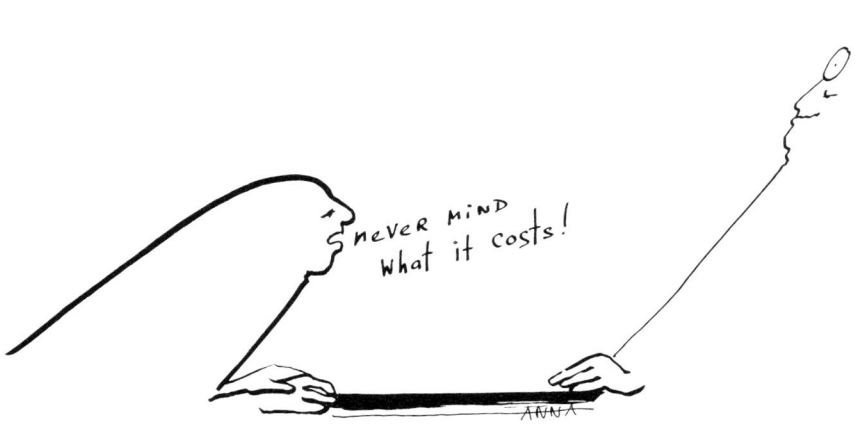

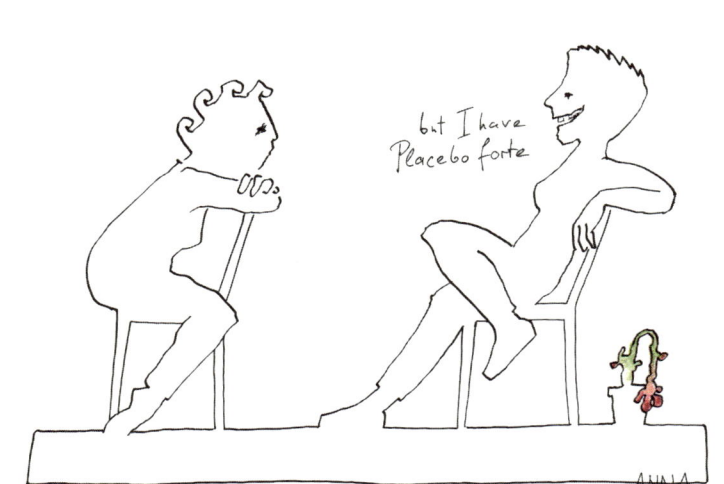

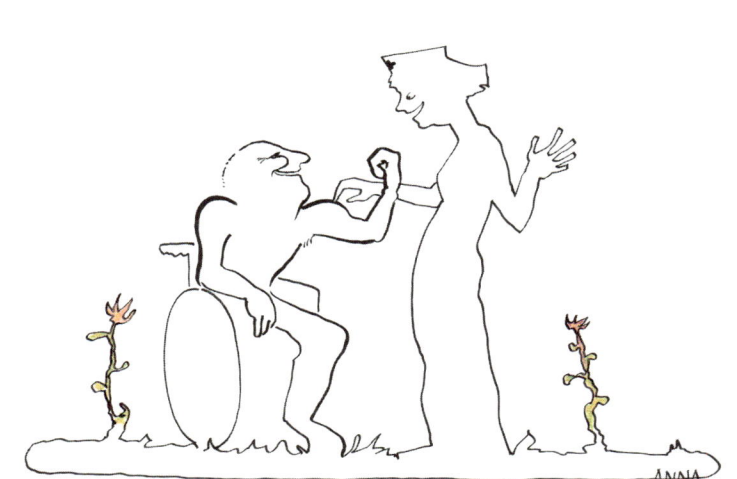

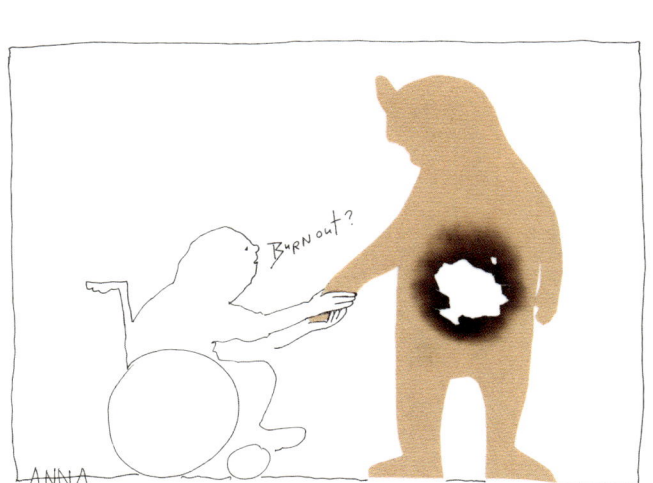

Publications:
"Wechseljahre" ["Menopause"] (Zytglogge-Verlag, 1997)
"1× täglich" ["1 per diem"], (Pharma Information/Zytglogge-Verlag, 1997)
"Inside outlandish", Tuttle, (Bergli Books, 1997)
"Lachfalten" ["Crow's Feet"] (Zytglogge-Verlag, 1998)
"Cordialement l'autre" (Editions Georg, 1999)
"ANNAlyse" (Schwabe & Co. AG, 2001)
informations: www.annahartmann.net

ISBN 3-905 252-03-1